FATTY LIVER DIET

COOKBOOK

DR. MAUREEN MOORE

CHAPTER ONE

Introduction

Welcome to the Fatty Liver Diet Cookbook, a comprehensive guide designed to support your journey towards a healthier liver and overall well-being. Fatty liver disease is a condition characterized by the accumulation of fat in the liver cells, which can lead to inflammation, scarring, and impaired liver function. Fortunately, adopting a balanced diet rich in nutrient-dense foods can play a crucial role in managing and even reversing this condition.

This cookbook is carefully crafted to provide you with delicious and nutritious recipes specifically tailored to support liver health. Whether you're newly diagnosed with fatty liver disease, seeking to prevent its progression, or simply aiming to optimize your liver function, the recipes and guidelines within these pages are here to empower you on your path to wellness.

The Role of Diet in Managing Fatty Liver Diet

Fortunately, adopting a liver-friendly diet can significantly impact the progression and management of fatty liver diet. By focusing on whole, nutrient-rich foods and avoiding or minimizing processed, sugary, and fatty foods, you can help reduce fat buildup in the liver, alleviate inflammation, and support overall liver function.

Key dietary principles for managing fatty liver diet cookbook include:

Emphasizing Plant-Based Foods: Vegetables, fruits, whole grains, legumes, nuts, and seeds are rich in vitamins, minerals, antioxidants, and fiber, all of which promote liver health and overall well-being.

Choosing Healthy Fats: Opt for sources of healthy fats such as avocados, olive oil, nuts, and fatty fish like salmon and mackerel, while limiting saturated and trans fats found in fried foods, processed snacks, and fatty meats.

Moderating Sugar and Refined Carbohydrates: Excessive sugar and refined carbs can contribute to insulin resistance and liver fat accumulation. Choose complex carbohydrates such as whole grains and legumes and limit added sugars and refined flour products.

Balancing Macronutrients: Aim for a balanced intake of carbohydrates, protein, and fat, with an emphasis on lean protein sources such as poultry, fish, tofu, and legumes.

Limiting Alcohol Consumption: If you have AFLD or NAFLD, it's essential to limit or eliminate alcohol consumption, as it can exacerbate liver damage and inflammation.

Principles of Fatty Liver Diet Cookbook

Emphasis on Whole, Nutrient-Dense Foods: The cookbook focuses on incorporating whole foods that are rich in nutrients such as vitamins, minerals, antioxidants, and fiber. These include fruits, vegetables, whole grains, legumes, lean proteins, and healthy fats. Whole foods provide essential nutrients that support liver health and overall well-being.

Limitation of Added Sugars and Refined Carbohydrates: The cookbook encourages minimizing the intake of added sugars and refined carbohydrates, as they can contribute to insulin resistance and liver fat accumulation. Instead, it promotes choosing complex carbohydrates and natural sources of sweetness, such as fruits and vegetables.

Inclusion of Healthy Fats: Healthy fats are an essential component of the Fatty Liver Diet Cookbook. It advocates for incorporating sources of healthy fats such as avocados, nuts, seeds, olive oil, and fatty fish like salmon and mackerel. These fats contain omega-3 fatty acids and other beneficial nutrients that help reduce inflammation and support liver function.

Moderation or Avoidance of Alcohol: If applicable, the cookbook advises limiting or abstaining from alcohol consumption, as it can exacerbate liver damage and inflammation. For individuals with alcoholic fatty liver disease or non-alcoholic fatty liver disease, reducing alcohol intake is essential for managing the condition and supporting liver health.

Balanced Macronutrient Intake: The cookbook promotes a balanced intake of carbohydrates, protein, and fat in each meal. It encourages incorporating lean proteins, complex carbohydrates, and healthy fats to create satisfying and nutritious meals that support liver health and overall wellness.

Portion Control and Mindful Eating: Portion control and mindful eating are emphasized throughout the cookbook to help individuals maintain a healthy weight and prevent overeating. By paying attention to portion sizes and listening to hunger and fullness cues, individuals can better manage their calorie intake and support their liver health.

Variety and Flavor: The cookbook offers a diverse array of recipes that are both nutritious and flavorful. From nourishing breakfasts and vibrant salads to hearty mains and indulgent desserts, there's something for every taste and occasion. By incorporating a variety of flavors, textures, and ingredients, individuals can enjoy delicious meals while supporting their liver health.

Education and Empowerment: In addition, to recipes, the cookbook provides practical tips, nutritional information, and meal planning guidance to educate and empower individuals to make informed choices about their diet and lifestyle. By understanding the principles of a Fatty Liver Diet Cookbook, individuals can take control of their health and well-being and make positive changes to support their liver health.

Benefits of Fatty Liver Diet Cookbook

Supports Liver Health: The primary benefit of a Fatty Liver Diet Cookbook is its focus on promoting liver health. By incorporating nutrient-dense foods and avoiding harmful dietary components, such as added sugars and excessive alcohol, the cookbook helps reduce liver fat accumulation, alleviate inflammation, and improve overall liver function.

Manages Fatty Liver Diet: For individuals already diagnosed with fatty liver disease, following a liver-friendly diet outlined in the cookbook can help manage the condition and prevent its progression to more severe stages, such as non-alcoholic steatohepatitis (NASH) or cirrhosis. By making appropriate dietary choices, individuals can potentially reverse liver damage and improve their prognosis.

Promotes Weight Management: Many of the dietary principles emphasized in the Fatty Liver Diet Cookbook, such as focusing on whole foods, limiting added sugars, and practicing portion control, support healthy weight management. Maintaining a healthy weight is crucial for individuals with fatty liver disease, as excess body weight and obesity are significant risk factors for the condition.

Improves Metabolic Health: By encouraging the consumption of nutrient-dense foods and healthy fats while limiting refined carbohydrates and unhealthy fats, the cookbook helps improve metabolic health. This includes better regulation of blood sugar levels, reduced insulin resistance, and lower levels of triglycerides in the blood, all of which are important for liver health and overall well-being.

Enhances Nutritional Status: The recipes featured in the Fatty Liver Diet Cookbook are designed to provide essential nutrients that support overall health and vitality. By incorporating a variety of fruits, vegetables, whole grains, lean proteins, and healthy fats, individuals can ensure they're meeting their nutritional needs while supporting their liver health.

Promotes Long-Term Lifestyle Changes: Unlike fad diets or temporary interventions, the Fatty Liver Diet Cookbook promotes sustainable lifestyle changes that individuals can maintain over the long term. By providing practical tips, meal planning guidance, and delicious recipes, the cookbook empowers individuals to make lasting improvements to their diet and lifestyle, leading to better health outcomes.

Guidelines of Fatty Liver Diet Cookbook

Consult with Healthcare Professionals: Before creating a Fatty Liver Diet Cookbook, it's essential to consult with healthcare professionals, such as registered dietitians, nutritionists, and hepatologists, who specialize in liver health. They can provide valuable insights, evidence-based recommendations, and guidance on dietary strategies for managing fatty liver diet.

Understand Target Audience: Understand the target audience for the cookbook, which may include individuals diagnosed with fatty liver disease, those at risk of developing the condition, caregivers, and healthcare professionals seeking resources for their patients. Tailor the content, recipes, and guidelines to meet the specific needs and preferences of the target audience.

Educate About Fatty Liver Diet: Include educational information about fatty liver diet, its causes, risk factors, symptoms, diagnosis, and potential complications. Provide an overview of the role of diet and lifestyle in managing the condition and empowering individuals to make informed choices about their health.

Focus on Nutrient-Dense Foods: Emphasize the importance of incorporating nutrient-dense foods into the diet, such as fruits, vegetables, whole grains, lean proteins, and healthy fats. Include a variety of colorful, flavorful ingredients to ensure a well-rounded and balanced diet that supports liver health and overall well-being.

Limit Added Sugars and Processed Foods: Encourage individuals to minimize their intake of added sugars, refined carbohydrates, and processed foods, which can contribute to liver fat accumulation and inflammation. Provide alternatives to common sources of added sugars and processed ingredients in recipes to promote healthier eating habits.

Include Liver-Friendly Recipes: Develop a collection of liver-friendly recipes that are delicious, nutritious, and easy to prepare. Include a variety of breakfasts, lunches, dinners, snacks, and desserts to accommodate different tastes and dietary preferences. Incorporate ingredients known for their liver-supportive properties, such as leafy greens, cruciferous vegetables, fatty fish, and nuts.

Provide Practical Tips and Guidelines: Offer practical tips, guidelines, and strategies for incorporating liver-friendly eating habits into daily life. This may include meal planning tips, portion control guidance, grocery shopping lists, cooking techniques, and suggestions for dining out or social occasions.

Promote Lifestyle Changes: Highlight the importance of adopting a holistic approach to managing fatty liver disease, which includes not only dietary changes but also regular physical activity, stress management, adequate sleep, and avoiding harmful habits such as excessive alcohol consumption and smoking.

Include Nutritional Information: Provide nutritional information for each recipe, including calories, macronutrients (carbohydrates, protein, fat), fiber, vitamins, minerals, and other relevant nutrients. This allows individuals to make informed decisions about their dietary intake and monitor their nutritional needs.

Empower and Motivate: Empower individuals to take control of their health and make positive changes to support their liver health and overall well-being. Offer encouragement, motivation, and support throughout the cookbook to inspire individuals to embrace a healthier lifestyle and enjoy the benefits of nutritious eating.

By following these guidelines, a Fatty Liver Diet Cookbook can serve as a valuable resource for individuals seeking to manage fatty liver disease, improve their liver health, and enhance their quality of life through wholesome and delicious meals.

CHAPTER TWO

RECIPES FOR FATTY LIVER DIET COOKBOOK

Recipe 1: Grilled Salmon with Avocado Salsa

Ingredients:

4 salmon fillets (about 6 ounces each)

2 ripe avocados, diced

1 small red onion, finely chopped

1 tomato, diced

1 jalapeño pepper, seeded and minced

Juice of 2 limes

2 tablespoons chopped cilantro

Salt and pepper to taste

Instructions:

Preheat the grill to medium-high heat.

Season the salmon fillets with salt and pepper.

In a bowl, combine the diced avocado, red onion, tomato, jalapeño pepper, lime juice, cilantro, salt, and pepper to make the salsa.

Grill the salmon fillets for 4-5 minutes per side, or until cooked through and flaky.

Serve the grilled salmon topped with the avocado salsa.

Benefits:

Salmon is rich in omega-3 fatty acids, which help reduce inflammation and support liver health.

Avocado provides healthy fats and fiber, while also adding creaminess to the salsa.

This dish is high in protein and low in carbohydrates, making it suitable for individuals managing fatty liver disease.

Cooking Time: 10-12 minutes

Recipe 2: Quinoa and Vegetable Stir-Fry

Ingredients:

1 cup quinoa, rinsed and drained

2 cups water or vegetable broth

2 tablespoons olive oil

2 cloves garlic, minced

1 small onion, chopped

1 bell pepper, sliced

1 zucchini, sliced

1 cup broccoli florets

1 cup sliced mushrooms

2 tablespoons low-sodium soy sauce or tamari

1 tablespoon rice vinegar

1 teaspoon sesame oil

Salt and pepper to taste

Optional: sliced green onions and sesame seeds for garnish

Instructions:

In a saucepan, combine the quinoa and water or vegetable broth. Bring to a boil, then reduce heat to low, cover, and simmer for 15-20 minutes, or until the quinoa is cooked and the liquid is absorbed.

In a large skillet or wok, heat the olive oil over medium-high heat. Add the garlic and onion, and cook for 2-3 minutes until fragrant.

Add the bell pepper, zucchini, broccoli, and mushrooms to the skillet. Stir-fry for 5-7 minutes, or until the vegetables are tender-crisp.

In a small bowl, whisk together the soy sauce, rice vinegar, and sesame oil. Pour the sauce over the vegetables and quinoa in the skillet, and toss to combine.

Season with salt and pepper to taste. Garnish with sliced green onions and sesame seeds, if desired.

Benefits:

Quinoa is a gluten-free whole grain that provides fiber and protein, helping to promote satiety and stabilize blood sugar levels.

The stir-fried vegetables are rich in vitamins, minerals, and antioxidants, supporting liver health and overall well-being.

This dish is low in saturated fat and cholesterol, making it heart-healthy and suitable for individuals with fatty liver disease.

Cooking Time: 25-30 minutes

Recipe 3: Baked Chicken with Roasted Vegetables

Ingredients:

4 boneless, skinless chicken breasts

2 tablespoons olive oil

2 cloves garlic, minced

1 teaspoon dried thyme

1 teaspoon dried rosemary

Salt and pepper to taste

2 cups chopped mixed vegetables (such as carrots, bell peppers, and Brussels sprouts)

1 tablespoon balsamic vinegar

Instructions:

Preheat the oven to 400°F (200°C).

In a small bowl, combine the olive oil, minced garlic, dried thyme, dried rosemary, salt, and pepper to make a marinade.

Place the chicken breasts in a baking dish and brush them with the marinade, coating evenly.

In a separate bowl, toss the chopped vegetables with the remaining marinade and spread them around the chicken breasts in the baking dish.

Drizzle the vegetables with balsamic vinegar.

Bake in the preheated oven for 25-30 minutes, or until the chicken is cooked through and the vegetables are tender.

Benefits:

Chicken is a lean source of protein that is low in saturated fat, making it an excellent choice for individuals with fatty liver disease.

The mixed vegetables provide an array of vitamins, minerals, and antioxidants, supporting liver health and overall nutrition.

This dish is simple to prepare and customizable based on personal preferences and seasonal produce availability.

Cooking Time: 25-30 minutes

Recipe 4: Turkey and Vegetable Lettuce Wraps

Ingredients:

1-pound ground turkey

1 tablespoon olive oil

2 cloves garlic, minced

1 small onion, diced

1 bell pepper, diced

1 cup shredded carrots

1 cup shredded cabbage

2 tablespoons low-sodium soy sauce or tamari

1 tablespoon rice vinegar

1 teaspoon sesame oil

Salt and pepper to taste

Butter lettuce leaves, for wrapping

Instructions:

Heat olive oil in a large skillet over medium heat. Add garlic and onion, and sauté until fragrant, about 2 minutes.

Add ground turkey to the skillet and cook until browned, breaking it up with a spoon.

Add bell pepper, shredded carrots, and shredded cabbage to the skillet. Cook until vegetables are tender-crisp.

In a small bowl, whisk together soy sauce, rice vinegar, and sesame oil. Pour over the turkey and vegetable mixture, and stir to combine.

Season with salt and pepper to taste. Serve the turkey and vegetable mixture in butter lettuce leaves as wraps.

Benefits:

Turkey is a lean source of protein that is lower in saturated fat compared to red meat, making it a healthier option for individuals with fatty liver disease.

Vegetables like bell peppers, carrots, and cabbage provide vitamins, minerals, and fiber, which support liver health and overall nutrition.

Lettuce wraps are a lighter alternative to traditional bread-based wraps, reducing overall calorie and carbohydrate intake.

Cooking Time: 20 minutes

Recipe 5: Lentil and Vegetable Soup

Ingredients:

1 cup dried lentils, rinsed and drained

4 cups vegetable broth

1 tablespoon olive oil

1 onion, chopped

2 carrots, diced

2 celery stalks, diced

2 cloves garlic, minced

1 teaspoon ground cumin

1 teaspoon paprika

1/2 teaspoon turmeric

Salt and pepper to taste

Fresh parsley, for garnish

Instructions:

In a large pot, heat olive oil over medium heat. Add chopped onion, carrots, and celery, and sauté until softened, about 5 minutes.

Add minced garlic, ground cumin, paprika, and turmeric to the pot. Cook for 1-2 minutes until fragrant.

Add dried lentils and vegetable broth to the pot. Bring to a boil, then reduce heat to low, cover, and simmer for 20-25 minutes, or until lentils are tender.

Season with salt and pepper to taste. Garnish with fresh parsley before serving.

Benefits:

Lentils are a rich source of plant-based protein, fiber, and folate, which support liver health and overall nutrition.

Vegetables like onions, carrots, celery, and garlic provide essential vitamins, minerals, and antioxidants, helping to reduce inflammation and promote liver health.

This hearty soup is filling, satisfying, and easy to prepare, making it a perfect option for busy weeknights.

Cooking Time: 30-35 minutes

Recipe 6: Eggplant Parmesan

Ingredients:

2 medium eggplants, sliced into rounds

2 eggs, beaten

1 cup whole wheat breadcrumbs

1/2 cup grated Parmesan cheese

2 cups marinara sauce (homemade or store-bought)

1 cup shredded mozzarella cheese

Fresh basil leaves, for garnish

Olive oil cooking spray

Instructions:

Preheat the oven to 400°F (200°C). Line a baking sheet with parchment paper and spray with olive oil cooking spray.

Dip eggplant slices into beaten eggs, then coat with whole wheat breadcrumbs mixed with grated Parmesan cheese.

Place coated eggplant slices on the prepared baking sheet in a single layer. Spray the tops with olive oil cooking spray.

Bake in the preheated oven for 20-25 minutes, flipping halfway through, until eggplant is golden brown and tender.

Spread marinara sauce evenly over the bottom of a baking dish. Arrange baked eggplant slices on top of the sauce. Top with shredded mozzarella cheese.

Bake for an additional 10-15 minutes, or until cheese is melted and bubbly.

Garnish with fresh basil leaves before serving.

Benefits:

Eggplant is low in calories and rich in fiber, vitamins, and minerals, making it a nutritious addition to a fatty liver diet.

Whole wheat breadcrumbs provide fiber and complex carbohydrates, which help promote satiety and stabilize blood sugar levels.

This lighter version of eggplant Parmesan is baked, not fried, reducing overall calorie and fat intake while still delivering delicious flavor and texture.

Cooking Time: 45-50 minutes

Recipe 7: Spinach and Feta Stuffed Chicken Breast

Ingredients:

4 boneless, skinless chicken breasts

2 cups fresh spinach leaves

1/2 cup crumbled feta cheese

2 cloves garlic, minced

1 tablespoon olive oil

Salt and pepper to taste

Toothpicks or kitchen twine

Instructions:

Preheat the oven to 375°F (190°C). Line a baking dish with parchment paper or lightly grease with olive oil.

Using a sharp knife, butterfly each chicken breast by slicing horizontally through the thickest part, without cutting all the way through.

In a skillet, heat olive oil over medium heat. Add minced garlic and spinach leaves, and cook until spinach is wilted, about 2-3 minutes. Remove from heat.

Stuff each chicken breast with spinach mixture and crumbled feta cheese. Use toothpicks or kitchen twine to secure the openings.

Season stuffed chicken breasts with salt and pepper to taste. Place them in the prepared baking dish.

Bake in the preheated oven for 25-30 minutes, or until chicken is cooked through and juices run clear.

Benefits:

Chicken breasts are a lean source of protein, while spinach provides vitamins, minerals, and antioxidants that support liver health.

Feta cheese adds creamy texture and tangy flavor without excessive saturated fat, making it a healthier alternative to heavier cheeses.

This dish is elegant enough for entertaining but easy enough for a weeknight meal, making it a versatile addition to the Fatty Liver Diet Cookbook.

Cooking Time: 30-35 minutes

Recipe 8: Mediterranean Chickpea Salad

Ingredients:

2 cans (15 ounces each) chickpeas, rinsed and drained

1 cucumber, diced

1 bell pepper, diced

1 pint cherry tomatoes, halved

1/2 red onion, thinly sliced

1/4 cup chopped fresh parsley

1/4 cup chopped fresh mint

1/4 cup crumbled feta cheese (optional)

1/4 cup Kalamata olives, pitted and sliced

Juice of 1 lemon

2 tablespoons extra virgin olive oil

Salt and pepper to taste

Instructions:

In a large bowl, combine chickpeas, cucumber, bell pepper, cherry tomatoes, red onion, parsley, mint, feta cheese (if using), and Kalamata olives.

In a small bowl, whisk together lemon juice, extra virgin olive oil, salt, and pepper to make the dressing.

Pour the dressing over the chickpea mixture and toss to combine, ensuring all ingredients are evenly coated.

Taste and adjust seasoning as needed. Serve chilled or at room temperature.

Benefits:

Chickpeas are a rich source of plant-based protein, fiber, and essential nutrients, supporting liver health and overall nutrition.

The Mediterranean-inspired ingredients, including fresh vegetables, herbs, olives, and olive oil, provide a wide array of vitamins, minerals, and antioxidants that promote heart and liver health.

This salad is light, refreshing, and packed with flavor, making it a perfect option for lunch, dinner, or a healthy side dish.

Cooking Time: 15 minutes

Recipe 9: Baked Cod with Lemon and Herbs

Ingredients:

4 cod fillets (about 6 ounces each)

2 tablespoons olive oil

2 cloves garlic, minced

Zest of 1 lemon

Juice of 1 lemon

1 tablespoon chopped fresh parsley

1 tablespoon chopped fresh dill

Salt and pepper to taste

Lemon slices for garnish

Instructions:

Preheat the oven to 400°F (200°C). Line a baking sheet with parchment paper or lightly grease with olive oil.

Place cod fillets on the prepared baking sheet. Drizzle with olive oil and sprinkle minced garlic over the top.

In a small bowl, combine lemon zest, lemon juice, chopped parsley, chopped dill, salt, and pepper. Pour the mixture over the cod fillets, ensuring they are evenly coated.

Place lemon slices on top of each cod fillet for added flavor and presentation.

Bake in the preheated oven for 12-15 minutes, or until cod is opaque and flakes easily with a fork.

Benefits:

Cod is a lean source of protein and a good source of omega-3 fatty acids, which support heart and liver health.

Fresh herbs like parsley and dill add vibrant flavor and are rich in vitamins, minerals, and antioxidants that promote overall well-being.

This baked cod recipe is quick, easy, and perfect for busy weeknights, providing a nutritious and delicious meal that the whole family will enjoy.

Cooking Time: 15-20 minutes

Recipe 10: Turkey and Black Bean Chili

Ingredients:

1 pound ground turkey

1 tablespoon olive oil

1 onion, chopped

2 cloves garlic, minced

1 bell pepper, diced

1 jalapeño pepper, seeded and minced

1 can (15 ounces) black beans, rinsed and drained

1 can (15 ounces) diced tomatoes

2 cups low-sodium chicken broth

2 teaspoons chili powder

1 teaspoon ground cumin

1/2 teaspoon paprika

Salt and pepper to taste

Optional toppings: chopped cilantro, sliced green onions, shredded cheese, plain Greek yogurt

Instructions:

In a large pot or Dutch oven, heat olive oil over medium heat. Add chopped onion, minced garlic, diced bell pepper, and minced jalapeño pepper. Sauté until vegetables are softened, about 5 minutes.

Add ground turkey to the pot and cook until browned, breaking it up with a spoon.

Stir in black beans, diced tomatoes, chicken broth, chili powder, ground cumin, paprika, salt, and pepper. Bring to a simmer.

Reduce heat to low and let the chili simmer for 20-25 minutes, stirring occasionally, until flavors are well combined and chili has thickened to your desired consistency.

Taste and adjust seasoning as needed. Serve hot, topped with optional toppings if desired.

Benefits:

Ground turkey provides lean protein and is lower in saturated fat compared to beef, making it a healthier option for individuals with fatty liver disease.

Black beans are high in fiber, protein, and essential nutrients, supporting liver health and promoting satiety.

This hearty and flavorful chili is a satisfying meal that can be customized with various toppings to suit individual tastes and preferences.

Cooking Time: 30-35 minutes

Recipe 11: Zucchini Noodles with Pesto and Cherry Tomatoes

Ingredients:

4 medium zucchini, spiralized into noodles

1 cup cherry tomatoes, halved

1/4 cup prepared pesto sauce (homemade or store-bought)

2 tablespoons grated Parmesan cheese (optional)

Fresh basil leaves, for garnish

Salt and pepper to taste

Instructions:

In a large skillet, heat olive oil over medium heat. Add spiralized zucchini noodles and cherry tomatoes to the skillet.

Sauté for 3-4 minutes, or until zucchini noodles are tender-crisp and cherry tomatoes are slightly softened.

Stir in prepared pesto sauce and toss to coat the zucchini noodles and cherry tomatoes evenly.

Season with salt and pepper to taste. Sprinkle grated Parmesan cheese over the top, if desired.

Garnish with fresh basil leaves before serving.

Benefits:

Zucchini noodles provide a low-carb, gluten-free alternative to traditional pasta, reducing overall calorie and carbohydrate intake.

Cherry tomatoes add sweetness and color to the dish while providing vitamins, minerals, and antioxidants that support liver health.

Pesto sauce made with basil, olive oil, garlic, and pine nuts is rich in flavor and heart-healthy fats, making it a delicious and nutritious addition to the Fatty Liver Diet Cookbook.

Cooking Time: 10 minutes

Recipe 12: Baked Sweet Potato Fries

Ingredients:

2 large sweet potatoes, peeled and cut into fries

2 tablespoons olive oil

1 teaspoon paprika

1/2 teaspoon garlic powder

1/2 teaspoon onion powder

1/4 teaspoon cayenne pepper (optional)

Salt and pepper to taste

Fresh parsley, for garnish

Instructions:

Preheat the oven to 425°F (220°C). Line a baking sheet with parchment paper or lightly grease with olive oil.

In a large bowl, toss sweet potato fries with olive oil, paprika, garlic powder, onion powder, cayenne pepper (if using), salt, and pepper until evenly coated.

Spread the seasoned sweet potato fries in a single layer on the prepared baking sheet, making sure they are not overcrowded.

Bake in the preheated oven for 20-25 minutes, flipping halfway through, until fries are golden brown and crispy.

Garnish with fresh parsley before serving.

Benefits:

Sweet potatoes are a nutrient-dense root vegetable rich in vitamins, minerals, and antioxidants, including beta-carotene, which supports liver health and overall well-being.

Baking sweet potato fries with olive oil instead of frying reduces overall calorie and fat intake while still delivering delicious flavor and crispy texture.

This healthier alternative to traditional fries is easy to prepare and makes a satisfying side dish or snack for any occasion.

Cooking Time: 25-30 minutes

Recipe 13: Broccoli and Cauliflower Salad with Greek Yogurt Dressing

Ingredients:

4 cups broccoli florets

4 cups cauliflower florets

1/4 cup plain Greek yogurt

2 tablespoons lemon juice

1 tablespoon Dijon mustard

1 tablespoon honey or maple syrup

2 cloves garlic, minced

Salt and pepper to taste

Optional toppings: chopped green onions, sliced almonds, dried cranberries

Instructions:

Steam broccoli and cauliflower florets until tender-crisp, about 5-7 minutes. Remove from heat and let cool.

In a small bowl, whisk together plain Greek yogurt, lemon juice, Dijon mustard, honey or maple syrup, minced garlic, salt, and pepper to make the dressing.

In a large bowl, combine steamed broccoli and cauliflower florets with Greek yogurt dressing, tossing until evenly coated.

Taste and adjust seasoning as needed. Serve chilled or at room temperature, topped with optional toppings if desired.

Benefits:

Broccoli and cauliflower are cruciferous vegetables rich in vitamins, minerals, and antioxidants that support liver health and promote detoxification.

Greek yogurt is a high-protein, probiotic-rich dairy product that adds creaminess and tangy flavor to the dressing, without excessive saturated fat or added sugars.

This refreshing salad is light, flavorful, and packed with nutrients, making it a perfect side dish for summer picnics, potlucks, or holiday gatherings.

Cooking Time: 15 minutes

Recipe 14: Turkey and Vegetable Meatballs

Ingredients:

1 pound ground turkey

1/2 cup grated zucchini

1/2 cup grated carrots

1/4 cup finely chopped onion

2 cloves garlic, minced

1/4 cup chopped fresh parsley

1/4 cup grated Parmesan cheese

1 egg, beaten

1/4 cup whole wheat breadcrumbs

Salt and pepper to taste

Olive oil cooking spray

Instructions:

Preheat the oven to 375°F (190°C). Line a baking sheet with parchment paper or lightly grease with olive oil cooking spray.

In a large bowl, combine ground turkey, grated zucchini, grated carrots, chopped onion, minced garlic, chopped parsley, grated Parmesan cheese, beaten egg, whole wheat breadcrumbs, salt, and pepper. Mix until well combined.

Shape the turkey mixture into meatballs, about 1 inch in diameter, and place them on the prepared baking sheet.

Spray the tops of the meatballs with olive oil cooking spray to help them brown evenly.

Bake in the preheated oven for 20-25 minutes, or until meatballs are cooked through and lightly browned on the outside.

Benefits:

Ground turkey is a lean source of protein that is lower in saturated fat compared to beef, making it a healthier option for individuals with fatty liver disease.

Grated zucchini and carrots add moisture, flavor, and extra nutrients to the meatballs, while also helping to stretch the meat mixture and reduce calorie and fat content.

These turkey and vegetable meatballs are versatile and can be served with whole grain pasta, zucchini noodles, or as an appetizer with a dipping sauce for a delicious and nutritious meal.

Cooking Time: 25-30 minutes

Recipe 15: Quinoa Stuffed Bell Peppers

Ingredients:

4 bell peppers, halved and seeds removed

1 cup cooked quinoa

1 can (15 ounces) black beans, rinsed and drained

1 cup corn kernels (fresh or frozen)

1 cup diced tomatoes

1/2 cup shredded cheddar cheese

2 tablespoons chopped fresh cilantro

1 teaspoon ground cumin

1/2 teaspoon chili powder

Salt and pepper to taste

Instructions:

Preheat the oven to 375°F (190°C). Lightly grease a baking dish with olive oil or cooking spray.

In a large bowl, combine cooked quinoa, black beans, corn kernels, diced tomatoes, shredded cheddar cheese, chopped cilantro, ground cumin, chili powder, salt, and pepper. Mix until well combined.

Stuff each bell pepper half with the quinoa mixture, pressing down gently to pack it in.

Place stuffed bell peppers in the prepared baking dish. Cover with aluminum foil.

Bake in the preheated oven for 25-30 minutes, or until bell peppers are tender and filling is heated through.

Remove foil and bake for an additional 5 minutes to melt the cheese and lightly brown the tops of the peppers.

Benefits:

Bell peppers are rich in vitamins, minerals, and antioxidants, especially vitamin C, which supports liver health and boosts the immune system.

Quinoa is a gluten-free whole grain that provides protein, fiber, and essential nutrients, making it a nutritious and filling option for individuals with fatty liver disease.

These quinoa stuffed bell peppers are colorful, flavorful, and satisfying, making them a perfect option for meatless Mondays or a healthy vegetarian meal.

Cooking Time: 30-35 minutes

Recipe 16: Asian-Inspired Beef and Broccoli Stir-Fry

Ingredients:

1 pound flank steak, thinly sliced against the grain

2 tablespoons low-sodium soy sauce or tamari

1 tablespoon cornstarch

2 tablespoons olive oil

3 cloves garlic, minced

1 inch piece fresh ginger, minced

4 cups broccoli florets

1 bell pepper, sliced

1/4 cup low-sodium beef broth or water

2 tablespoons oyster sauce

1 tablespoon hoisin sauce

1 teaspoon sesame oil

Optional garnish: sliced green onions, sesame seeds

Instructions:

In a bowl, combine sliced flank steak with low-sodium soy sauce and cornstarch. Toss until evenly coated and set aside to marinate for 15-20 minutes.

Heat olive oil in a large skillet or wok over medium-high heat. Add minced garlic and ginger, and sauté for 1-2 minutes until fragrant.

Add marinated flank steak to the skillet in a single layer. Cook for 2-3 minutes without stirring to allow the meat to sear and brown on one side.

Add broccoli florets and sliced bell pepper to the skillet. Stir-fry for an additional 3-4 minutes, or until vegetables are tender-crisp and beef is cooked to your desired doneness.

In a small bowl, whisk together low-sodium beef broth or water, oyster sauce, hoisin sauce, and sesame oil. Pour the sauce over the beef and vegetables in the skillet.

Cook for 1-2 minutes, stirring constantly, until the sauce thickens and coats the beef and vegetables evenly.

Garnish with sliced green onions and sesame seeds before serving.

Benefits:

Flank steak is a lean cut of beef that provides high-quality protein and essential nutrients, including iron and zinc, which support liver health and overall well-being.

Broccoli is rich in vitamins, minerals, and antioxidants that help reduce inflammation and support detoxification processes in the liver.

This Asian-inspired beef and broccoli stir-fry is quick, easy, and packed with flavor, making it a perfect option for busy weeknights when you need a nutritious and satisfying meal in a hurry.

Cooking Time: 20-25 minutes

Recipe 17: Greek Chicken Souvlaki

Ingredients:

1 pound boneless, skinless chicken breasts, cut into cubes

2 tablespoons olive oil

2 cloves garlic, minced

1 teaspoon dried oregano

1 teaspoon dried thyme

Juice of 1 lemon

Salt and pepper to taste

Wooden skewers, soaked in water for at least 30 minutes

Tzatziki sauce for serving (optional)

Instructions:

In a bowl, combine olive oil, minced garlic, dried oregano, dried thyme, lemon juice, salt, and pepper to make the marinade.

Add cubed chicken breasts to the marinade and toss until evenly coated. Cover and refrigerate for at least 30 minutes to allow the flavors to meld.

Preheat the grill or grill pan over medium-high heat.

Thread marinated chicken cubes onto soaked wooden skewers, leaving a little space between each piece.

Grill the chicken skewers for 6-8 minutes per side, or until cooked through and lightly charred on the outside.

Serve hot with tzatziki sauce for dipping, if desired.

Benefits:

Chicken breasts are a lean source of protein that is low in saturated fat, making them an excellent choice for individuals with fatty liver disease.

The marinade made with olive oil, garlic, lemon juice, and herbs adds flavor and moisture to the chicken, while also providing heart-healthy fats and antioxidants.

This Greek chicken souvlaki recipe is simple, flavorful, and perfect for summer grilling, providing a taste of the Mediterranean without compromising liver health.

Cooking Time: 15-20 minutes

Recipe 18: Spaghetti Squash with Turkey Bolognese Sauce

Ingredients:

1 medium spaghetti squash

1 tablespoon olive oil

1 pound ground turkey

1 onion, chopped

2 cloves garlic, minced

1 carrot, grated

1 celery stalk, diced

1 can (15 ounces) crushed tomatoes

1 tablespoon tomato paste

1 teaspoon dried basil

1 teaspoon dried oregano

Salt and pepper to taste

Fresh parsley, for garnish

Grated Parmesan cheese (optional)

Instructions:

Preheat the oven to 400°F (200°C). Line a baking sheet with parchment paper.

Cut the spaghetti squash in half lengthwise and scoop out the seeds. Brush the cut sides with olive oil and place them cut-side down on the prepared baking sheet.

Roast the spaghetti squash in the preheated oven for 40-45 minutes, or until tender when pierced with a fork. Let cool slightly.

While the spaghetti squash is roasting, prepare the turkey bolognese sauce. Heat olive oil in a large skillet over medium heat. Add ground turkey and cook until browned, breaking it up with a spoon.

Add chopped onion, minced garlic, grated carrot, and diced celery to the skillet. Sauté until vegetables are softened, about 5 minutes.

Stir in crushed tomatoes, tomato paste, dried basil, dried oregano, salt, and pepper. Simmer for 15-20 minutes, stirring occasionally, until flavors are well combined and sauce has thickened.

Use a fork to scrape the flesh of the roasted spaghetti squash into strands. Divide the spaghetti squash among serving plates and top with turkey bolognese sauce.

Garnish with fresh parsley and grated Parmesan cheese, if desired.

Benefits:

Spaghetti squash is a low-carb, nutrient-dense alternative to traditional pasta, providing fiber, vitamins, and minerals that support liver health and overall well-being.

Ground turkey is a lean source of protein that is lower in saturated fat compared to beef, making it a healthier option for individuals with fatty liver disease.

This spaghetti squash with turkey bolognese sauce is a satisfying and flavorful meal that's perfect for cozy weeknight dinners or entertaining guests with dietary restrictions.

Cooking Time: 60-65 minutes

Recipe 19: Mediterranean Chickpea and Vegetable Stew

Ingredients:

2 tablespoons olive oil

1 onion, chopped

2 cloves garlic, minced

1 bell pepper, diced

1 zucchini, diced

1 eggplant, diced

1 can (15 ounces) chickpeas, rinsed and drained

1 can (15 ounces) diced tomatoes

2 cups vegetable broth

1 teaspoon dried oregano

1 teaspoon dried basil

Salt and pepper to taste

Fresh parsley, for garnish

Crumbled feta cheese (optional)

Instructions:

Heat olive oil in a large pot or Dutch oven over medium heat. Add chopped onion and minced garlic, and sauté until fragrant, about 2 minutes.

Add diced bell pepper, diced zucchini, and diced eggplant to the pot. Cook for 5-7 minutes, or until vegetables are softened.

Stir in chickpeas, diced tomatoes, vegetable broth, dried oregano, dried basil, salt, and pepper. Bring to a simmer.

Reduce heat to low and let the stew simmer for 20-25 minutes, stirring occasionally, until flavors are well combined and vegetables are tender.

Taste and adjust seasoning as needed. Serve hot, garnished with fresh parsley and crumbled feta cheese, if desired.

Benefits:

Chickpeas are a rich source of plant-based protein, fiber, and essential nutrients, supporting liver health and promoting satiety.

The Mediterranean-inspired combination of vegetables, including bell peppers, zucchini, and eggplant, provides vitamins, minerals, and antioxidants that reduce inflammation and support liver function.

This hearty and flavorful stew is easy to prepare and perfect for meal prep, providing a nutritious and satisfying meal that can be enjoyed throughout the week.

Cooking Time: 35-40 minutes

Recipe 20: Asian-Inspired Tofu Stir-Fry

Ingredients:

1 block (14 ounces) extra-firm tofu, pressed and cubed

2 tablespoons low-sodium soy sauce or tamari

1 tablespoon cornstarch

2 tablespoons sesame oil, divided

2 cloves garlic, minced

1 inch piece fresh ginger, minced

2 cups mixed vegetables (such as bell peppers, broccoli, carrots, snap peas)

1/4 cup low-sodium vegetable broth

2 tablespoons hoisin sauce

1 tablespoon rice vinegar

1 teaspoon honey or maple syrup

Optional garnish: sliced green onions, sesame seeds

Instructions:

In a bowl, combine cubed tofu with low-sodium soy sauce and cornstarch. Toss until evenly coated and set aside.

Heat 1 tablespoon of sesame oil in a large skillet or wok over medium-high heat. Add minced garlic and ginger, and sauté for 1-2 minutes until fragrant.

Add marinated tofu cubes to the skillet in a single layer. Cook for 3-4 minutes on each side, or until golden brown and crispy. Remove tofu from the skillet and set aside.

Heat the remaining tablespoon of sesame oil in the same skillet. Add mixed vegetables and stir-fry for 5-7 minutes, or until tender-crisp.

In a small bowl, whisk together low-sodium vegetable broth, hoisin sauce, rice vinegar, and honey or maple syrup to make the sauce.

Return cooked tofu to the skillet with the vegetables. Pour the sauce over the tofu and vegetables, tossing to coat evenly.

Cook for 1-2 minutes, stirring constantly, until the sauce thickens and coats the tofu and vegetables.

Garnish with sliced green onions and sesame seeds before serving.

Benefits:

Tofu is a versatile plant-based protein source that is rich in protein, calcium, and iron, making it an excellent choice for individuals following a vegetarian or vegan diet.

Mixed vegetables provide a wide array of vitamins, minerals, and antioxidants that support liver health and overall well-being.

This Asian-inspired tofu stir-fry is quick, easy, and packed with flavor, making it a perfect option for meatless Mondays or a delicious and nutritious weeknight meal.

Cooking Time: 20-25 minutes

Recipe 21: Salmon and Asparagus Foil Packets

Ingredients:

4 salmon fillets (about 6 ounces each)

1-pound asparagus spears, trimmed

2 tablespoons olive oil

2 cloves garlic, minced

Zest of 1 lemon

Juice of 1 lemon

1 teaspoon dried dill

Salt and pepper to taste

Lemon slices for garnish

Instructions:

Preheat the oven to 400°F (200°C). Cut four large pieces of aluminum foil.

Place a salmon fillet in the center of each piece of foil. Arrange asparagus spears around the salmon.

In a small bowl, whisk together olive oil, minced garlic, lemon zest, lemon juice, dried dill, salt, and pepper. Drizzle the mixture over the salmon and asparagus.

Fold the edges of the foil over the salmon and asparagus to create a packet, sealing tightly.

Place the foil packets on a baking sheet and bake in the preheated oven for 15-20 minutes, or until salmon is cooked through and flakes easily with a fork.

Carefully open the foil packets and transfer the salmon and asparagus to serving plates. Garnish with lemon slices before serving.

Benefits:

Salmon is rich in omega-3 fatty acids, which support heart and liver health, while asparagus provides vitamins, minerals, and antioxidants that promote detoxification and reduce inflammation.

Cooking salmon and asparagus in foil packets helps lock in moisture and flavor while minimizing cleanup, making it a convenient and delicious option for weeknight dinners.

Cooking Time: 20-25 minutes

Recipe 22: Quinoa and Black Bean Stuffed Bell Peppers

Ingredients:

4 bell peppers, halved and seeds removed

1 cup cooked quinoa

1 can (15 ounces) black beans, rinsed and drained

1 cup corn kernels (fresh or frozen)

1 cup diced tomatoes

1/2 cup shredded cheddar cheese

2 tablespoons chopped fresh cilantro

1 teaspoon ground cumin

1/2 teaspoon chili powder

Salt and pepper to taste

Instructions:

Preheat the oven to 375°F (190°C). Lightly grease a baking dish with olive oil or cooking spray.

In a large bowl, combine cooked quinoa, black beans, corn kernels, diced tomatoes, shredded cheddar cheese, chopped cilantro, ground cumin, chili powder, salt, and pepper. Mix until well combined.

Stuff each bell pepper half with the quinoa mixture, pressing down gently to pack it in.

Place stuffed bell peppers in the prepared baking dish. Cover with aluminum foil.

Bake in the preheated oven for 25-30 minutes, or until bell peppers are tender and filling is heated through.

Remove foil and bake for an additional 5 minutes to melt the cheese and lightly brown the tops of the peppers.

Benefits:

Quinoa is a gluten-free whole grain that provides protein, fiber, and essential nutrients, making it a nutritious and filling option for individuals with fatty liver disease.

Black beans are rich in fiber, protein, and antioxidants, supporting liver health and promoting satiety.

These quinoa and black bean stuffed bell peppers are colorful, flavorful, and satisfying, making them a perfect option for meatless meals or a healthy vegetarian entree.

Cooking Time: 30-35 minutes

Recipe 23: Baked Chicken Parmesan

Ingredients:

4 boneless, skinless chicken breasts

1/2 cup whole wheat breadcrumbs

1/4 cup grated Parmesan cheese

1 teaspoon dried Italian seasoning

1/2 teaspoon garlic powder

1/2 teaspoon onion powder

Salt and pepper to taste

1 egg, beaten

Olive oil cooking spray

1 cup marinara sauce (homemade or store-bought)

1/2 cup shredded mozzarella cheese

Fresh basil leaves, for garnish

Instructions:

Preheat the oven to 400°F (200°C). Line a baking sheet with parchment paper or lightly grease with olive oil cooking spray.

In a shallow dish, combine whole wheat breadcrumbs, grated Parmesan cheese, dried Italian seasoning, garlic powder, onion powder, salt, and pepper.

Dip each chicken breast into the beaten egg, then coat with the breadcrumb mixture, pressing gently to adhere.

Place breaded chicken breasts on the prepared baking sheet. Spray the tops with olive oil cooking spray.

Bake in the preheated oven for 20-25 minutes, or until chicken is cooked through and golden brown.

Remove chicken from the oven and top each breast with marinara sauce and shredded mozzarella cheese.

Return to the oven and bake for an additional 5-7 minutes, or until cheese is melted and bubbly.

Garnish with fresh basil leaves before serving.

Benefits:

Chicken breasts are a lean source of protein that is lower in saturated fat compared to red meat, making them a healthier option for individuals with fatty liver disease.

Whole wheat breadcrumbs provide fiber and complex carbohydrates, which help promote satiety and stabilize blood sugar levels.

This baked chicken Parmesan recipe is lighter than the traditional fried version, reducing overall calorie and fat intake while still delivering delicious flavor and texture.

Cooking Time: 30-35 minutes

Recipe 24: Shrimp and Vegetable Stir-Fry

Ingredients:

1 pound large shrimp, peeled and deveined

2 tablespoons low-sodium soy sauce or tamari

1 tablespoon cornstarch

2 tablespoons olive oil, divided

2 cloves garlic, minced

1 inch piece fresh ginger, minced

2 cups mixed vegetables (such as bell peppers, broccoli, carrots, snap peas)

1/4 cup low-sodium chicken broth or water

1 tablespoon hoisin sauce

1 teaspoon sesame oil

1/2 teaspoon crushed red pepper flakes (optional)

Optional garnish: sliced green onions, sesame seeds

Instructions:

In a bowl, combine peeled and deveined shrimp with low-sodium soy sauce and cornstarch. Toss until evenly coated and set aside.

Heat 1 tablespoon of olive oil in a large skillet or wok over medium-high heat. Add minced garlic and ginger, and sauté for 1-2 minutes until fragrant.

Add marinated shrimp to the skillet in a single layer. Cook for 2-3 minutes on each side, or until pink and opaque. Remove shrimp from the skillet and set aside.

Heat the remaining tablespoon of olive oil in the same skillet. Add mixed vegetables and stir-fry for 5-7 minutes, or until tender-crisp.

In a small bowl, whisk together low-sodium chicken broth or water, hoisin sauce, sesame oil, and crushed red pepper flakes (if using) to make the sauce.

Return cooked shrimp to the skillet with the vegetables. Pour the sauce over the shrimp and vegetables, tossing to coat evenly.

Cook for 1-2 minutes, stirring constantly, until the sauce thickens and coats the shrimp and vegetables.

Garnish with sliced green onions and sesame seeds before serving.

Benefits:

Shrimp is a low-calorie source of protein that is rich in omega-3 fatty acids, which support heart and liver health.

Mixed vegetables provide vitamins, minerals, and antioxidants that help reduce inflammation and promote detoxification processes in the liver.

This shrimp and vegetable stir-fry is quick, easy, and packed with flavor, making it a perfect option for busy weeknights when you need a nutritious and satisfying meal in a hurry.

Cooking Time: 20-25 minutes

Recipe 25: Lentil and Vegetable Soup

Ingredients:

1 tablespoon olive oil

1 onion, chopped

2 carrots, diced

2 celery stalks, diced

2 cloves garlic, minced

1 cup dried green or brown lentils, rinsed and drained

1 can (15 ounces) diced tomatoes

4 cups low-sodium vegetable broth

2 cups water

1 teaspoon dried thyme

1 teaspoon dried rosemary

Salt and pepper to taste

Fresh parsley, for garnish

Instructions:

Heat olive oil in a large pot or Dutch oven over medium heat. Add chopped onion, diced carrots, and diced celery. Sauté until vegetables are softened, about 5 minutes.

Add minced garlic to the pot and sauté for an additional 1-2 minutes until fragrant.

Stir in rinsed and drained lentils, diced tomatoes, vegetable broth, water, dried thyme, dried rosemary, salt, and pepper. Bring to a simmer.

Reduce heat to low and let the soup simmer for 30-35 minutes, or until lentils are tender and flavors are well combined.

Taste and adjust seasoning as needed. Serve hot, garnished with fresh parsley.

Benefits:

Lentils are a rich source of plant-based protein, fiber, and essential nutrients, supporting liver health and promoting satiety.

This lentil and vegetable soup is packed with vitamins, minerals, and antioxidants from the vegetables and herbs, providing immune-boosting and anti-inflammatory benefits.

Enjoy this hearty and comforting soup as a nutritious and satisfying meal for lunch or dinner, especially during colder months when you crave something warm and nourishing.

Cooking Time: 35-40 minutes

Recipe 26: Turkey and Spinach Meatballs

Ingredients:

1 pound ground turkey

1/2 cup whole wheat breadcrumbs

1/4 cup grated Parmesan cheese

1/4 cup chopped fresh parsley

2 cloves garlic, minced

1/2 teaspoon dried oregano

1/2 teaspoon dried basil

Salt and pepper to taste

1 egg, beaten

Olive oil cooking spray

Instructions:

Preheat the oven to 400°F (200°C). Line a baking sheet with parchment paper or lightly grease with olive oil cooking spray.

In a large bowl, combine ground turkey, whole wheat breadcrumbs, grated Parmesan cheese, chopped fresh parsley, minced garlic, dried oregano, dried basil, salt, pepper, and beaten egg. Mix until well combined.

Shape the turkey mixture into meatballs, about 1 inch in diameter, and place them on the prepared baking sheet.

Spray the tops of the meatballs with olive oil cooking spray to help them brown evenly.

Bake in the preheated oven for 15-20 minutes, or until meatballs are cooked through and lightly browned on the outside.

Benefits:

Ground turkey is a lean source of protein that is lower in saturated fat compared to beef, making it a healthier option for individuals with fatty liver disease.

Spinach adds moisture, flavor, and extra nutrients to the meatballs, while also contributing to their vibrant green color.

These turkey and spinach meatballs are versatile and can be served with whole grain pasta, zucchini noodles, or as an appetizer with a dipping sauce for a delicious and nutritious meal.

Cooking Time: 20-25 minutes

Recipe 27: Eggplant Parmesan

Ingredients:

2 medium eggplants, sliced into 1/2-inch rounds

Salt

1 cup whole wheat breadcrumbs

1/4 cup grated Parmesan cheese

1 teaspoon dried Italian seasoning

1/2 teaspoon garlic powder

1/2 teaspoon onion powder

Salt and pepper to taste

2 eggs, beaten

Olive oil cooking spray

2 cups marinara sauce (homemade or store-bought)

1 cup shredded mozzarella cheese

Fresh basil leaves, for garnish

Instructions:

Place eggplant slices in a colander and sprinkle with salt. Let sit for 20-30 minutes to draw out excess moisture. Rinse and pat dry with paper towels.

Preheat the oven to 400°F (200°C). Line a baking sheet with parchment paper or lightly grease with olive oil cooking spray.

In a shallow dish, combine whole wheat breadcrumbs, grated Parmesan cheese, dried Italian seasoning, garlic powder, onion powder, salt, and pepper.

Dip each eggplant slice into beaten eggs, then coat with the breadcrumb mixture, pressing gently to adhere.

Place breaded eggplant slices on the prepared baking sheet. Spray the tops with olive oil cooking spray.

Bake in the preheated oven for 20-25 minutes, flipping halfway through, until eggplant is golden brown and crispy.

Remove eggplant from the oven and reduce oven temperature to 350°F (175°C).

In a baking dish, spread a thin layer of marinara sauce. Arrange half of the baked eggplant slices in the dish, overlapping slightly.

Top eggplant slices with more marinara sauce and shredded mozzarella cheese. Repeat with remaining eggplant slices, marinara sauce, and mozzarella cheese.

Bake in the oven for 20-25 minutes, or until cheese is melted and bubbly.

Garnish with fresh basil leaves before serving.

Benefits:

Eggplant is a low-calorie vegetable that is rich in fiber, vitamins, and minerals, supporting liver health and promoting satiety.

Baking eggplant instead of frying reduces overall calorie and fat intake while still delivering delicious flavor and texture.

This eggplant Parmesan recipe is a healthier twist on the classic Italian dish, making it a satisfying and nutritious meal for lunch or dinner.

Cooking Time: 45-50 minutes

Recipe 28: Cauliflower Fried Rice

Ingredients:

1 head cauliflower, riced (or 4 cups store-bought cauliflower rice)

2 tablespoons olive oil

2 eggs, beaten

2 cloves garlic, minced

1-inch piece fresh ginger, minced

1 cup mixed vegetables (such as peas, carrots, bell peppers)

2 tablespoons low-sodium soy sauce or tamari

2 green onions, sliced

Salt and pepper to taste

Instructions:

If using a whole head of cauliflower, cut it into florets and pulse in a food processor until it resembles rice. Alternatively, use store-bought cauliflower rice.

Heat 1 tablespoon of olive oil in a large skillet or wok over medium heat. Add beaten eggs and scramble until cooked through. Remove scrambled eggs from the skillet and set aside.

Heat the remaining tablespoon of olive oil in the same skillet. Add minced garlic and ginger, and sauté for 1-2 minutes until fragrant.

Add mixed vegetables to the skillet and stir-fry for 3-4 minutes, or until tender-crisp.

Add riced cauliflower to the skillet and cook for 5-7 minutes, stirring frequently, until cauliflower is cooked through but still slightly crisp.

Return cooked eggs to the skillet with the cauliflower and vegetables. Drizzle with low-sodium soy sauce or tamari and toss to coat evenly.

Cook for an additional 1-2 minutes, stirring constantly, until everything is heated through.

Season with salt and pepper to taste. Garnish with sliced green onions before serving.

Benefits:

Cauliflower is a low-calorie, nutrient-dense vegetable that is rich in fiber, vitamins, and minerals, supporting liver health and promoting satiety.

Using cauliflower rice instead of traditional rice reduces overall calorie and carbohydrate intake, making this dish suitable for individuals with fatty liver disease or those following a low-carb diet.

This cauliflower fried rice recipe is quick, easy, and customizable, making it a perfect option for busy weeknights when you need a nutritious and satisfying meal in a hurry.

Cooking Time: 20-25 minutes

Recipe 29: Greek Quinoa Salad

Ingredients:

1 cup cooked quinoa

1 cup cherry tomatoes, halved

1 cucumber, diced

1 bell pepper, diced

1/4 cup diced red onion

1/4 cup chopped fresh parsley

1/4 cup crumbled feta cheese

2 tablespoons Kalamata olives, sliced

2 tablespoons olive oil

1 tablespoon lemon juice

1 teaspoon dried oregano

Salt and pepper to taste

Instructions:

In a large bowl, combine cooked quinoa, cherry tomatoes, cucumber, bell pepper, red onion, chopped parsley, crumbled feta cheese, and sliced Kalamata olives.

In a small bowl, whisk together olive oil, lemon juice, dried oregano, salt, and pepper to make the dressing.

Pour the dressing over the quinoa salad and toss until evenly coated.

Taste and adjust seasoning as needed. Serve chilled or at room temperature.

Benefits:

Quinoa is a gluten-free whole grain that provides protein, fiber, and essential nutrients, making it a nutritious and filling option for individuals with fatty liver disease.

Cherry tomatoes, cucumber, bell pepper, red onion, and parsley add color, flavor, and extra nutrients to the salad, while feta cheese and Kalamata olives provide a salty and tangy kick.

This Greek quinoa salad is light, refreshing, and packed with Mediterranean flavors, making it a perfect side dish or light lunch for any occasion.

Cooking Time: 15 minutes

Recipe 30: Turkey and Vegetable Chili

Ingredients:

1 tablespoon olive oil

1 onion, chopped

2 cloves garlic, minced

1-pound ground turkey

1 bell pepper, diced

1 zucchini, diced

1 carrot, diced

1 can (15 ounces) diced tomatoes

1 can (15 ounces) kidney beans, rinsed and drained

1 cup low-sodium chicken broth

2 tablespoons tomato paste

1 tablespoon chili powder

1 teaspoon ground cumin

1 teaspoon paprika

Salt and pepper to taste

Optional toppings: shredded cheddar cheese, chopped green onions, Greek yogurt

Instructions:

Heat olive oil in a large pot or Dutch oven over medium heat. Add chopped onion and minced garlic, and sauté until fragrant, about 2 minutes.

Add ground turkey to the pot and cook until browned, breaking it up with a spoon.

Stir in diced bell pepper, diced zucchini, and diced carrot. Cook for 5-7 minutes, or until vegetables are softened.

Add diced tomatoes, kidney beans, low-sodium chicken broth, tomato paste, chili powder, ground cumin, paprika, salt, and pepper. Stir to combine.

Bring the chili to a simmer, then reduce heat to low and let it simmer for 20-25 minutes, stirring occasionally, until flavors are well combined and vegetables are tender.

Taste and adjust seasoning as needed. Serve hot, garnished with shredded cheddar cheese, chopped green onions, and a dollop of Greek yogurt if desired.

Benefits:

Ground turkey is a lean source of protein that is lower in saturated fat compared to beef, making it a healthier option for individuals with fatty liver disease.

This turkey and vegetable chili is packed with fiber, vitamins, and minerals from the vegetables and beans, supporting liver health and promoting satiety.

Enjoy this hearty and flavorful chili as a nutritious and satisfying meal for lunch or dinner, especially during colder months when you crave something warm and comforting.

Cooking Time: 30-35 minutes

These recipes offer a diverse range of flavors, textures, and nutrients while supporting liver health and overall well-being. Enjoy experimenting with these delicious and nutritious meals from the Fatty Liver Diet Cookbook!

CONCLUSION

In conclusion, the Fatty Liver Diet Cookbook offers a comprehensive collection of delicious and nutritious recipes designed to support liver health and overall well-being. From vibrant salads to comforting soups, flavorful stir-fries to hearty stews, each recipe is carefully crafted to provide a balance of essential nutrients while minimizing saturated fats, refined sugars, and processed ingredients.

By incorporating ingredients rich in antioxidants, vitamins, minerals, and fiber, these recipes promote detoxification, reduce inflammation, and support optimal liver function. Whether you're following a specific dietary plan for managing fatty liver disease or simply aiming to make healthier food choices, the diverse range of options in this cookbook ensures that there's something for everyone.

So, dive into the world of flavorful dishes and discover how simple, wholesome ingredients can transform your meals and elevate your well-being. Whether you're a novice in the kitchen or a seasoned chef, the Fatty Liver Diet Cookbook is your companion on the journey to a healthier, happier you. Here's to good food, good health, and good living!